DO YOU SOMETIMES NEED TO SWEAR BUT CAN'T?

DOES IT ANNOY THE SHITAKE MUSHROOM OUT OF YOU?

WELL THEN THIS BOOK IS PERFECT!

EACH PAGE IN THIS BOOK HAS A RELAXING MANDALA CONTAINING A CLEAN SWEAR WORD THAT YOU CAN USE AS OFTEN AS YOU LIKE!

HAPPY COLORING!

Copyright © 2018 Coloring Crew.
All rights reserved.
ISBN-13: 978-1987431582
ISBN-10: 1987431588

COLORING CREW

COLORING CREW

COLORING CREW

COLORING CREW

COLORING CREW

COLORING CREW

COLORING CREW

COLORING CREW

COLORING CREW

COLORING CREW

COLORING CREW

COLORING CREW

COLORING CREW

COLORING CREW

COLORING CREW

COLORING CREW

COLORING CREW

COLORING CREW

COLORING CREW

COLORING CREW

COLORING CREW

THANKS!
WE HOPE YOU HAD FUN!

IF YOU LIKED THIS BOOK THEN YOU YOU CAN VIEW OUR FULL RANGE OF HILARIOUS ADULT COLORING BOOKS BY GOING TO AMAZON AND SEARCHING FOR "COLORING CREW" AND THEN CLICKING ON OUR AUTHOR PAGE.

THANKS AGAIN!

COLORING CREW

www.ingramcontent.com/pod-product-compliance
Lightning Source LLC
Chambersburg PA
CBHW062126220526
45471CB00010B/3892